Vakarė Rimkutė

Lymphatic Diet Cookbook: Uncovering Lymphatic Wellness Secrets Through Nutritious, Delicious, and Satisfying Culinary Creations.

Dedicated to the brave lymphatic patients, may this cookbook nourish your healing journey, one delicious recipe at a time." Your courage inspires us, and this book is a gesture of our support for your wellness journey.

Contents

1.

2.

   1.

   2.

   3.

3.

   1.

   2.

   3.

4.

   1.

   2.

   3.

5.

   1.

2.

3.

6.

1.

2.

3.

7.

1.

2.

3.

8.

1.

2.

3.

9.

1.

2.

3.

10.

Preface

Thank You For Picking Up This Cookbook.

In the journey towards health and vitality, we often seek ways to nourish our bodies and uplift our spirits. At times, life throws unexpected challenges our way, and one such challenge that some of us face is a compromised lymphatic system. The lymphatic system, that unsung hero, quietly working behind the scenes to support our overall well-being, may need a little extra attention and care. It's in response to this need that the "Lymphatic Diet Cookbook" comes to life.

This cookbook is more than simply a recipe collection; it is an invitation to go on a transforming path toward improved health. It's an acceptance of the concept that food can be medicine and that by eating mindfully, we can cultivate our lymphatic system and, in turn, nurture our entire selves.

If you're reading this, you're probably already on your way to lymphatic well-being, or you're just getting started. Regardless matter where you are on your path, the "Lymphatic Diet Cookbook" is a reliable friend. It exists to motivate, educate, and empower you to take charge of your health.

This book is a labour of love, written with sensitivity and compassion for people dealing with lymphatic issues. We gathered the help of specialists in nutrition, medicine, and lymphatic health to compile a selection of dishes that are not only tasty but also high in the nutrients your lymphatic system requires. Each meal is carefully prepared to adhere to the principles of the lymphatic diet while still being delicious and flavorful.

This cookbook, however, is more than just a compilation of recipes. It's a manual for living well. You'll discover helpful hints on meal planning, navigating grocery store aisles, and information on the need for hydration and detoxification. We've also included particular sections for dietary problems such as gluten sensitivity, vegan and vegetarian options, and allergen-free recipes since we think that excellent health should be available to everyone.

Aside from the recipes and dietary advice, this book serves as a reminder that you are not alone on your path. You are part of a community of people who understand your struggles and are committed to improving their well-being. The "Lymphatic Diet Cookbook" is a monument to your fortitude and perseverance.

We invite you to embrace this gastronomic and health trip with an open heart and an open mind. Accept the flavours, relish the textures, and take pleasure in the act of fueling your body. By doing so, you are actively participating in your healing process.

This book is for you, the lymphatic sufferer who wants to flourish rather than merely endure. It is dedicated to the families and friends who have provided unflinching support. It is intended for caregivers, healthcare professionals, and curious individuals interested in learning more about the lymphatic system and its tremendous influence on human health.

Thank you for allowing the "Lymphatic Diet Cookbook" to into your life. May it serve as a source of inspiration, hope, and empowerment for you. We can begin on a health journey together, one delicious, lymphatic-friendly food at a time.

With our warmest wishes for your good health,

Vakarė   Rimkutė

Chapter 1: Introduction to the Lymphatic Diet

What exactly is the Lymphatic System?

The lymphatic system is a complex network of tissues, organs, veins, and fluids that plays an important part in the general health and immunological function of the body. It is a parallel circulatory system to the blood circulatory system, and its primary function is to convey lymph, a clear, colourless fluid containing white blood cells and waste materials.

The lymphatic system's main components and functions are as follows:

1. **Nodes Lymphatic**: Lymph nodes are little bean-shaped structures found all over the body. They function as filters, capturing and eliminating bacteria, viruses, and other potentially hazardous items from the lymph. Lymph nodes are essential for immune system function and play a role in infection defence.

2. **Lymphatic vessels**: are a network of tiny tubes that transport lymph throughout the body. They serve to maintain fluid

balance and eliminate waste items by transporting lymph from various tissues and organs back into circulation.

3. **Lymphatic Fluid (Lymph)**: Lymph is a fluid generated from plasma in the blood. It is made up of white blood cells (lymphocytes), which are necessary for immunological responses. Lymphs also transport proteins, lipids, and trash.

4. **Lymphatic Organs:** The lymphatic system comprises lymphoid organs such as the spleen, thymus, and tonsils in addition to lymph nodes. These organs aid in immune function by filtering and processing lymph.

5. **Bone Marrow:** The bone marrow is in charge of creating white blood cells, including lymphocytes. Lymphocytes play an important role in the body's defence against infections and illnesses.

6. **Tonsils and Adenoids:** are lymphoid tissue clusters found in the throat. They aid in the prevention of infections that enter the body through the mouth and nose.

The lymphatic system performs various critical activities, including:

1. **Immunological Function**: It filters and destroys dangerous things such as bacteria, viruses, and damaged cells as part of the body's immunological response. Lymphocytes are an important part of the immune system.

2. **Fluid Balance**: The lymphatic system aids in the maintenance of fluid balance in the body. It gathers extra fluid that escapes from blood arteries and returns it to

circulation, preventing fluid buildup in tissues, which can cause swelling (oedema).

3. **Nutrient Absorption**: The lymphatic system is involved in the absorption of dietary lipids and fat-soluble vitamins in the small intestine, delivering them to the circulation.

4. **Waste Removal:** The lymphatic system transports waste products and cellular debris from the body, assisting in detoxification.

The Importance of Having a Healthy Lymphatic System:

A healthy lymphatic system is critical to sustaining general health and well-being. Here are some of the main reasons why a healthy lymphatic system is essential:

1. **Immunological Defense:** The lymphatic system is a critical component of the body's immunological defence. Lymph nodes are found all across the body and serve as filters for dangerous things such as bacteria, viruses, and aberrant cells. They are the sites where white blood cells (lymphocytes) are created and activated to fight infections. A healthy lymphatic system improves the body's ability to fight infections and illnesses.

2. **Detoxification**: The lymphatic system is essential for removing waste and toxins from the body. It gathers cellular

waste, surplus fluids, and debris, assisting in the detoxification of tissues and the maintenance of a healthy interior environment.

3. **Fluid Balance:** The lymphatic system aids in the maintenance of fluid balance in the body. It catches extra fluid that seeps from blood arteries, avoiding oedema (swelling). This function is crucial in controlling tissue fluid and blood volume.

4. **Nutrient Absorption:** The lymphatic system in the digestive system is in charge of absorbing dietary lipids and fat-soluble vitamins. These nutrients are delivered to the circulation via lymphatic veins, facilitating adequate nutritional use by the organism.

5. **Lipid Transport**: The lymphatic system carries and distributes lipids (fats) absorbed from the digestive system to the circulation. This is necessary for energy production and the support of many body activities.

6. **Wound Healing**: The lymphatic system aids in wound healing by eliminating debris and excess fluid from the site of damage. It promotes tissue regeneration and healing.

7. When tissues become inflamed as a result of injury or infection, the lymphatic system assists in controlling the inflammatory process by emptying excess fluid and white blood cells from the afflicted region.

8. **Maintaining Homeostasis:** A healthy lymphatic system contributes to the body's general homeostasis, which is the balance and stability of internal circumstances required for good health.

9. **Lymphedema**: is a disorder characterized by swelling, most typically in the arms or legs, caused by a weakened lymphatic system. A healthy lymphatic system can aid in the prevention or management of this illness.

The lymphatic diet's fundamental concepts are as follows:

The lymphatic diet is a dietary strategy aimed at promoting and maintaining the health of the lymphatic system, which is an important component of the immunological and circulatory systems of the body. The lymphatic system filters and transports lymph, a fluid containing white blood cells and waste materials, throughout the body.

While there is no conventional lymphatic diet, the following basic ideas are usually connected with it:

1. **Hydration**: A healthy lymphatic system requires adequate hydration. Drinking enough water helps to maintain the flow of lymph and ensures that the system operates properly. Drinking filtered water, herbal teas, and other hydration liquids is emphasized in several lymphatic diet guidelines.

2. **Low Sodium**: A basic tenet of the lymphatic diet is to limit sodium consumption. High sodium levels can cause water retention and oedema, putting extra strain on the lymphatic

system. The diet frequently supports the use of low-sodium meals to preserve good lymphatic function.

3. **Entire Foods**: The lymphatic diet emphasizes entire, unadulterated foods. Whole grains, lean proteins, fruits, and vegetables are promoted as nutrient-dense foods with fewer amounts of additives, preservatives, and salt than processed meals.

4. **Foods with Anti-Inflammatory characteristics**: Many lymphatic diets include foods with anti-inflammatory characteristics. This can assist to minimize inflammation in the lymphatic system, which is essential for its healthy function. Berries, leafy greens, and fatty fish (high in omega-3 fatty acids) are frequently included.

5. **Lymphatic-Supporting Ingredients**: Some foods and herbs are considered to support lymphatic health, and these are typically integrated into the diet. Parsley, ginger, turmeric, and citrus fruits are among examples.

6. **Low Sugar:** A lymphatic diet might include a reduction in refined sugar intake. High sugar consumption can contribute to inflammation, which can have a harmful influence on the lymphatic system. Natural fruit sugars are favoured over artificial sugars.

7. Eating in moderation is suggested to avoid overloading the lymphatic system with extra calories and waste materials. Proper portion management can also aid in the maintenance of a healthy weight, which is essential for lymphatic health.

8. Exercise and physical exercise regularly are thought to be good for the lymphatic system. Yoga, rebounding (using a

little trampoline), and walking may be suggested to help with lymphatic circulation.

9. **Consideration for Supplements:** Some lymphatic diet regimens include supplements such as vitamin C and antioxidants to assist in boosting the immune system and reducing inflammation.

Chapter 2: Breakfast Recipes

Nutrient-rich smoothies:

Recipe 1: Green Superfood Smoothie

Ingredients:

- 1 cup spinach or kale (or a combination of both)
- 1/2 cup frozen berries (such as blueberries or strawberries)
- 1/2 banana
- 1 tablespoon chia seeds
- 1 tablespoon flaxseeds
- 1/2 cup Greek yoghurt or a dairy-free alternative
- 1 cup unsweetened almond milk (or your preferred milk)
- Honey or maple syrup for sweetness (optional)

Instructions:

1. Add the spinach or kale, frozen berries, banana, chia seeds, flaxseeds, Greek yoghurt, and almond milk to a blender.
2. If desired, add a drizzle of honey or maple syrup for sweetness.
3. Blend until the mixture is smooth and creamy. You may need to stop and scrape down the sides of the blender to ensure everything is well-mixed.

4. Pour the smoothie into a glass and enjoy immediately.

Recipe 2: Tropical Immunity Booster

Ingredients:

- 1/2 cup pineapple chunks
- 1/2 cup mango chunks
- 1 small orange, peeled and segmented
- 1/2 cup Greek yoghurt or coconut yoghurt
- 1 tablespoon honey (optional)
- 1/2 cup water or coconut water

Instructions:

1. Place the pineapple chunks, mango chunks, orange segments, Greek yoghurt, and water (or coconut water) in a blender.
2. Add honey for sweetness if desired.
3. Blend until the mixture is smooth and creamy.
4. Pour the smoothie into a glass and savour the tropical flavours.

Lymphatic-friendly oatmeal:

Ingredients:

- 1/2 cup old-fashioned rolled oats
- 1 cup almond milk (or any non-dairy milk of your choice)
- 1/4 cup fresh berries (blueberries, strawberries, raspberries)

- 1 tablespoon chia seeds
- 1 tablespoon flax seeds
- 1/2 teaspoon ground cinnamon
- 1/4 teaspoon grated fresh ginger
- 1/4 teaspoon turmeric powder
- 1 tablespoon raw honey or maple syrup (optional for sweetness)
- Sliced almonds or walnuts for garnish (optional)
- Fresh mint leaves for garnish (optional)

Instructions:

1. **Combine Oats and Liquid**: In a saucepan, combine the rolled oats and almond milk. Stir well.

2. **Add Spices and Herbs**: Add the cinnamon, grated ginger, and turmeric powder to the oats. These spices have anti-inflammatory properties that can benefit the lymphatic system. Stir to combine.

3. **Heat and Cook**: Place the saucepan over medium heat and cook, stirring frequently, until the oatmeal reaches your desired consistency. This usually takes about 5-7 minutes.

4. **Stir in Seeds**: Remove the saucepan from the heat, and stir in the chia seeds and flax seeds. These seeds are rich in fibre and healthy fats, which can support digestion and detoxification.

5. **Sweeten, If Desired**: If you prefer your oatmeal to be sweeter, you can add a drizzle of raw honey or maple syrup. Adjust the sweetness to your taste.

6. **Top with Berries**: Serve the oatmeal in a bowl and top it with fresh berries. Berries are packed with antioxidants that can help reduce inflammation.
7. **Garnish**: Optionally, garnish your lymphatic-friendly oatmeal with sliced almonds or walnuts for added texture and healthy fats. You can also add a few fresh mint leaves for a burst of flavour

Basic Fresh Fruit Salad:

Ingredients:

- 2 cups of fresh strawberries, hulled and halved
- 1 cup of fresh blueberries
- 1 cup of fresh pineapple, diced
- 1 cup of fresh grapes (red or green), halved
- 1 large orange, peeled and segmented
- 1 banana, sliced
- 2 tablespoons of honey (or maple syrup for a vegan option)
- 1 tablespoon of freshly squeezed lemon juice
- Optional: Fresh mint leaves for garnish

Instructions:

1. Wash and prepare the fruits as needed. Ensure that they are all cut into bite-sized pieces.

2. In a large mixing bowl, combine the strawberries, blueberries, pineapple, grapes, orange segments, and banana slices.

3. In a separate small bowl, whisk together the honey and freshly squeezed lemon juice to create the dressing.

4. Drizzle the dressing over the fruit in the mixing bowl.

5. Gently toss the fruit and dressing together until the fruits are evenly coated.

6. Taste the fruit salad and adjust the sweetness or acidity as needed by adding more honey or lemon juice.

7. If desired, garnish the fruit salad with fresh mint leaves.

8. Serve the fresh fruit salad immediately or refrigerate for a short time before serving for a chilled option.

Chapter 3: Lunch Recipes

Lymphatic-Boosting Citrus Salad:

Ingredients:

- 2 cups mixed greens (spinach, arugula, and romaine)
- 1 orange, peeled and segmented
- 1/2 grapefruit, peeled and segmented
- 1/4 cup sliced cucumber
- 1/4 cup fresh berries (blueberries or strawberries)
- 1/4 avocado, diced
- Balsamic vinaigrette dressing

Instructions:

1. Place the mixed greens in a salad bowl.
2. Add the orange and grapefruit segments, cucumber slices, fresh berries, and diced avocado.
3. Drizzle with balsamic vinaigrette dressing.
4. Toss gently to combine, and serve immediately.

Lymphatic-Boosting Kale Salad

Ingredients:

- 3 cups chopped kale
- 1/4 cup diced cucumber
- 1/4 cup cherry tomatoes, halved
- 1/4 cup sliced red bell pepper
- 1/4 cup sliced strawberries
- 1/4 cup crumbled feta cheese (optional)
- Lemon-tahini dressing

Instructions:

1. Massage the kale with a little olive oil to soften it.
2. Add the cucumber, cherry tomatoes, red bell pepper, and strawberries.
3. If desired, sprinkle crumbled feta cheese on top.
4. Drizzle with lemon-tahini dressing.
5. Toss to combine, and enjoy.

Light soups and broths:

Vegetable Clear Broth: This clear vegetable broth is simple to make and soothing for the body. It's perfect for when you want something light and nutritious.

Ingredients:

- 4 cups of vegetable broth (homemade or store-bought)

- 1 carrot, thinly sliced
- 1 celery stalk, thinly sliced
- 1 small onion, finely chopped
- 1 clove garlic, minced
- 1/2 cup of green beans, chopped
- 1/2 cup of peas (fresh or frozen)
- Salt and pepper to taste
- Fresh parsley for garnish (optional)

Instructions:

1. In a large pot, heat a little olive oil over medium heat. Add the chopped onion, celery, and carrot. Sauté for a few minutes until they begin to soften.
2. Add the minced garlic and continue to sauté for another minute or until fragrant.
3. Pour in the vegetable broth and bring it to a boil. Reduce the heat and let it simmer for about 10-15 minutes.
4. Add the green beans and peas to the broth. Cook for an additional 5-7 minutes or until the vegetables are tender.
5. Season the broth with salt and pepper to taste. You can also add fresh parsley for garnish if desired.

Chicken and Rice Soup: This chicken and rice soup is another example of a light and comforting option. It's easy on the stomach and provides essential nutrients.

Ingredients:

- 4 cups of chicken broth
- 1 boneless, skinless chicken breast
- 1/2 cup of white rice
- 1 carrot, diced
- 1 celery stalk, diced
- 1/2 small onion, finely chopped
- Salt and pepper to taste
- Fresh dill or parsley for garnish (optional)

Instructions:

1. In a pot, bring the chicken broth to a boil. Add the chicken breast and simmer for about 15-20 minutes or until the chicken is cooked through.
2. Remove the chicken breast from the broth, shred it with a fork, and set it aside.
3. Add the diced carrot, celery, and onion to the broth. Cook for 10-15 minutes or until the vegetables are tender.
4. Add the white rice and continue to simmer for another 15 minutes or until the rice is cooked.
5. Return the shredded chicken to the soup, and season with salt and pepper to taste.
6. Garnish with fresh dill or parsley if desired.

Grilled vegetable platters:

Basic Grilled Vegetable Platter Recipe:

Ingredients:

- Assorted vegetables (e.g., bell peppers, zucchini, eggplant, tomatoes, onions, asparagus, mushrooms)
- Olive oil
- Salt and pepper
- Fresh herbs (e.g., rosemary, thyme, or basil) for garnish
- Balsamic vinegar or lemon juice for drizzling (optional)

Instructions:

1. **Preparation**:
- Wash and dry the vegetables.
- Cut the vegetables into uniform-sized pieces to ensure even cooking.

2. **Marinade**:
- In a bowl, mix olive oil, salt, and pepper to create a simple marinade. You can add minced garlic or herbs for additional flavour.

3. **Coat the Vegetables:**
- Toss the vegetables in the marinade, ensuring they are evenly coated.

4. Preheat the Grill:

- Preheat your grill to medium-high heat.

5. Grilling:

- Place the vegetables directly on the grill grates or use a grill basket or skewers for smaller pieces.

- Grill the vegetables until they have grill marks and are tender but not overcooked. Cooking times may vary depending on the vegetable; for example, bell peppers and zucchini cook faster than denser vegetables like potatoes.

- Rotate or flip the vegetables as needed to cook them evenly.

6. Arrange on a Platter:

- Once the vegetables are grilled to your liking, remove them from the grill and arrange them on a serving platter.

7. Garnish:

- Sprinkle fresh herbs over the grilled vegetables for added freshness and flavour.

8. Optional Drizzle:

- Drizzle balsamic vinegar or lemon juice over the platter to enhance the flavours.

9. Serve:

- Serve the grilled vegetable platter as a side dish, appetizer, or main   course.

Chapter 4: Dinner Recipes

Grilled Lemon Herb Chicken:

Ingredients:

- 4 boneless, skinless chicken breasts
- 2 tablespoons olive oil
- 2 tablespoons lemon juice
- 2 cloves garlic, minced
- 1 teaspoon dried oregano
- 1 teaspoon dried thyme
- Salt and pepper to taste

Instructions:

1. In a bowl, whisk together the olive oil, lemon juice, minced garlic, dried oregano, dried thyme, salt, and pepper.
2. Place the chicken breasts in a zip-top bag or a shallow dish and pour the marinade over them. Seal the bag or cover the dish and refrigerate for at least 30 minutes, or up to 4 hours for the best flavor.
3. Preheat your grill to medium-high heat.

4. Remove the chicken from the marinade and grill for about 6-8 minutes per side, or until the internal temperature reaches 165°F (75°C) and the chicken is no longer pink in the centre.

5. Serve the grilled lemon herb chicken with your choice of side dishes, such as a fresh salad or steamed vegetables.

Whole grain dishes:

Quinoa Salad:

Ingredients:

- 1 cup quinoa
- 2 cups water or vegetable broth
- Various chopped vegetables (bell peppers, cucumbers, cherry tomatoes, etc.)
- Fresh herbs (parsley, mint, cilantro)
- Olive oil and lemon juice dressing
- Feta cheese (optional)

Instructions:

1. Rinse quinoa thoroughly and cook it with water or vegetable broth according to package instructions.
2. Fluff the cooked quinoa with a fork and let it cool.
3. Toss the quinoa with chopped vegetables, herbs, and dressing.

4. Add feta cheese if desired.

5. Serve chilled.

Brown Rice and Vegetable Stir-Fry:

Ingredients:

- 1 cup brown rice
- 2 cups water
- Assorted stir-fry vegetables (bell peppers, broccoli, carrots, snap peas)
- Tofu or chicken (optional)
- Stir-fry sauce (soy sauce, ginger, garlic, and honey)

Instructions:

1. Cook brown rice according to package instructions.
2. In a pan, stir-fry your choice of protein (tofu or chicken) until cooked and set aside.
3. Stir-fry the vegetables in the same pan until they're tender.
4. Add the cooked protein back to the pan and mix with the vegetables.
5. Pour the stir-fry sauce over the mixture and cook for a few more minutes.
6. Serve the stir-fry over brown rice.

Barley and Mushroom Risotto:

Ingredients:

- 1 cup pearl barley
- 4 cups vegetable broth
- 2 cups sliced mushrooms
- Onion and garlic, chopped
- White wine (optional)
- Parmesan cheese (optional)

Instructions:

1. Sauté onions and garlic in a pan until translucent.
2. Add the sliced mushrooms and cook until they release their moisture.
3. Stir in the pearl barley and cook for a few minutes.
4. If using, deglaze the pan with white wine and cook until it's mostly evaporated.
5. Add vegetable broth gradually, stirring frequently until the barley is tender and creamy.
6. If desired, stir in Parmesan cheese.
7. Season with salt and pepper and serve.

Whole Wheat Pasta with Pesto:

Ingredients:

- Whole wheat pasta
- Fresh basil pesto (homemade or store-bought)
- Cherry tomatoes

- Pine nuts
- Grated Parmesan cheese

Instructions:

1. Cook the whole wheat pasta according to package instructions.
2. Drain the pasta and toss it with fresh basil pesto.
3. Add halved cherry tomatoes and toasted pine nuts.
4. Top with grated Parmesan cheese and serve.

Low-sodium recipes:

Herb-Roasted Chicken with Vegetables

Ingredients:

- 4 boneless, skinless chicken breasts
- 4 cups mixed vegetables (e.g., carrots, broccoli, bell peppers)
- 2 tablespoons olive oil
- 2 cloves garlic, minced
- 1 tablespoon fresh rosemary, chopped
- 1 tablespoon fresh thyme, chopped
- Salt-free herb seasoning (available in stores)
- Ground black pepper to taste

Instructions:

1. Preheat the oven to 375°F (190°C).
2. In a large bowl, toss the vegetables with olive oil, minced garlic, and salt-free herb seasoning.
3. Season the chicken breasts with the chopped rosemary and thyme, along with a dash of ground black pepper.
4. Place the chicken and vegetables in a baking dish and roast for 25-30 minutes or until the chicken is cooked through and the vegetables are tender.

Lemon and Dill Baked Salmon

Ingredients:

- 4 salmon fillets
- 2 tablespoons fresh lemon juice
- 2 teaspoons fresh dill, chopped
- 1 teaspoon olive oil
- 1/2 teaspoon garlic powder
- Ground black pepper to taste

Instructions:

1. Preheat the oven to 375°F (190°C).
2. Place salmon fillets in a baking dish.
3. In a small bowl, mix lemon juice, dill, olive oil, garlic powder, and ground black pepper.
4. Pour the lemon-dill mixture over the salmon fillets.

5. Bake for about 15-20 minutes or until the salmon flakes easily with a fork.

Quinoa and Black Bean Salad

Ingredients:

- 1 cup quinoa
- 2 cups water
- 1 can (15 oz) black beans, drained and rinsed
- 1 cup corn kernels (fresh or frozen)
- 1 red bell pepper, diced
- 1/4 cup fresh cilantro, chopped
- Dressing: 2 tablespoons fresh lime juice, 2 tablespoons olive oil, and ground black pepper to taste

Instructions:

1. Rinse quinoa thoroughly and cook it according to the package instructions, using water.
2. In a large bowl, combine the cooked quinoa, black beans, corn, red bell pepper, and cilantro.
3. In a separate small bowl, whisk together the lime juice, olive oil, and ground black pepper.
4. Drizzle the dressing over the quinoa mixture and toss to combine.

Chapter 5: Snacks and Appetizers

Lymphatic-friendly dips and spreads:

Cucumber and Greek Yogurt Dip:

Ingredients:

- 1 cup Greek yogurt
- 1/2 cucumber, finely grated and drained
- 1 clove garlic, minced
- 1 tablespoon fresh dill, chopped
- Salt and pepper to taste

Instructions:

1. In a bowl, combine the Greek yoghurt, grated cucumber, minced garlic, and chopped dill.
2. Mix well and season with salt and pepper to taste.
3. Refrigerate for about 30 minutes before serving with fresh vegetable sticks.

Avocado and Spinach Spread:

Ingredients:

- 1 ripe avocado
- 1 cup fresh spinach, blanched and chopped
- 2 cloves garlic, minced
- Juice of 1/2 lemon
- Salt and pepper to taste

Instructions:

1. Mash the ripe avocado in a bowl.
2. Add the blanched and chopped spinach, minced garlic, and lemon juice.
3. Season with salt and pepper to taste.
4. Mix until well combined. Serve on whole-grain crackers or as a sandwich spread.

Roasted Red Pepper Hummus:

Ingredients:

- 1 can (15 oz) chickpeas, drained and rinsed
- 2 roasted red peppers (from a jar or freshly roasted)
- 2 tablespoons tahini
- 2 cloves garlic, minced
- Juice of 1 lemon
- 2 tablespoons olive oil
- Salt and paprika to taste

Instructions:

1. In a food processor, combine the chickpeas, roasted red peppers, tahini, minced garlic, lemon juice, and olive oil.
2. Blend until smooth. If the mixture is too thick, add a little water to achieve the desired consistency.
3. Season with salt and paprika to taste. Refrigerate and serve with raw vegetable sticks.

Nut and seed mixes:

Recipe 1: Sweet and Savory Nut and Seed Mix

Ingredients:

- 1 cup almonds
- 1/2 cup pumpkin seeds
- 1/2 cup sunflower seeds
- 1/2 cup dried cranberries
- 1 tablespoon olive oil
- 1 tablespoon honey or maple syrup
- 1/2 teaspoon sea salt
- 1/4 teaspoon ground cinnamon

Instructions:

1. Preheat your oven to 325°F (163°C).

2. In a bowl, combine the almonds, pumpkin seeds, and sunflower seeds.

3. In a separate small bowl, mix the olive oil, honey or maple syrup, sea salt, and ground cinnamon.

4. Pour the liquid mixture over the nut and seed mixture and stir to coat evenly.

5. Spread the mixture evenly on a baking sheet lined with parchment paper.

6. Roast in the oven for about 15-20 minutes, stirring occasionally, until the nuts and seeds are lightly toasted.

7. Allow the mixture to cool, then add the dried cranberries and toss to combine.

8. Store in an airtight container.

Recipe 2: Spicy Nut and Seed Mix

Ingredients:

- 1 cup mixed nuts (almonds, cashews, peanuts)
- 1/2 cup sesame seeds
- 1/4 cup pumpkin seeds
- 1 tablespoon olive oil
- 1 teaspoon chilli powder
- 1/2 teaspoon paprika
- 1/4 teaspoon cayenne pepper
- 1/2 teaspoon sea salt

Instructions:

1. In a large bowl, combine the mixed nuts, sesame seeds, and pumpkin seeds.
2. In a separate small bowl, mix the olive oil, chilli powder, paprika, cayenne pepper, and sea salt.
3. Pour the spicy mixture over the nuts and seeds, and toss to coat them evenly.
4. Spread the mixture on a baking sheet and bake in a preheated oven at 325°F (163°C) for about 15-20 minutes, stirring occasionally until the nuts are toasted and fragrant.
5. Allow the mix to cool before storing it in an airtight container.

Fresh veggie platters:

Ingredients:

- Carrot sticks
- Celery sticks
- Cherry tomatoes
- Cucumber slices
- Bell pepper strips (various colours)
- Broccoli florets
- Cauliflower florets
- Snap peas or sugar snap peas

- Radishes (sliced)
- Baby carrots
- Your choice of dip (e.g., hummus, Greek yoghurt-based dip, or a low-fat ranch dressing)

Instructions:

1. Wash all the vegetables thoroughly, and if needed, peel and cut them into bite-sized pieces or sticks. Arrange them on a large serving platter, leaving space in the centre for your chosen dip.

2. In the centre of the platter, place a small bowl or dish filled with your preferred dip. You can choose from various options like hummus, a Greek yoghurt-based dip with herbs and spices, or a low-fat ranch dressing.

3. Arrange the vegetables on the platter appealingly and colourfully. You can organize them in rows or create a beautiful pattern. The more colourful and varied the veggies, the more visually appealing your platter will be.

4. Serve the fresh veggie platter as an appetizer, snack, or a side dish. You can refrigerate it if you're making it in advance, but it's best served fresh to retain the crispness of the veggies.

5. Enjoy your fresh veggie platter by dipping the vegetables into your chosen dip. It's a great way to increase your daily intake of vegetables while keeping your lymphatic diet on track.

Chapter 6: Desserts and Sweets

Fruit-based desserts:

F**ruit Salad:**

Ingredients:

- Assorted fresh fruits (e.g., strawberries, blueberries, kiwi, pineapple, mango, grapes, etc.)
- A drizzle of honey or a splash of citrus juice for added flavor

Instructions:

1. Wash and chop the fruits into bite-sized pieces.
2. Combine the fruits in a large bowl.
3. Optionally, drizzle with honey or citrus juice for added sweetness and flavour.
4. Toss gently to mix the fruits, and refrigerate before serving.

Baked Apples:

Ingredients:

- Apples (choose sweet varieties like Fuji or Honeycrisp)

- Cinnamon
- A touch of honey (optional)
- Chopped nuts (e.g., walnuts or almonds) for added crunch (optional)

Instructions:

1. Preheat the oven to 375°F (190°C).
2. Core the apples and remove the seeds.
3. Sprinkle each apple with cinnamon and, if desired, drizzle with honey.
4. Place the apples in a baking dish and bake for about 20-25 minutes until they are soft.
5. Optionally, top with chopped nuts before serving.

Berry Parfait:

Ingredients:

- Greek yoghurt or dairy-free alternative
- Fresh or frozen mixed berries (e.g., strawberries, blueberries, raspberries)
- Granola or crushed nuts
- Honey for drizzling (optional)

Instructions:

1. In a glass or bowl, layer Greek yoghurt, mixed berries, and granola.

2. Repeat the layers until you've filled the container.

3. Optionally, drizzle honey over the top for sweetness.

Grilled Peaches:

Ingredients:

- Ripe peaches, halved and pitted
- Olive oil for brushing
- Honey for drizzling
- Greek yoghurt or ice cream (optional)

Instructions:

1. Preheat a grill or grill pan to medium-high heat.
2. Brush the peach halves with a little olive oil.
3. Grill the peaches for about 2-3 minutes per side until they have grill marks and are tender.
4. Drizzle honey over the grilled peaches and serve with a scoop of Greek yoghurt or a small portion of ice cream.

Low-Sugar Treat Recipes:

Berry Yogurt Parfait:

Ingredients:

- 1 cup Greek yogurt

- 1/2 cup mixed berries (e.g., strawberries, blueberries, raspberries)
- 1 tablespoon honey or maple syrup (adjust to taste)
- 1/4 cup granola (optional)

Instructions:

- In a bowl, mix the Greek yoghurt and honey or maple syrup.
- In a glass or bowl, layer the yoghurt mixture, mixed berries, and granola (if using) in repeating layers.
- Serve immediately or refrigerate for a refreshing low-sugar dessert or snack.

Dark Chocolate-Covered Almonds:

Ingredients:

- 1 cup raw almonds
- 4 oz dark chocolate (70% cocoa or higher)

Instructions:

- Melt the dark chocolate in a microwave or on a stovetop using a double boiler.
- Dip the almonds into the melted chocolate, ensuring they are well coated.
- Place the chocolate-covered almonds on a parchment paper-lined tray and allow them to cool and harden.

- Once the chocolate has set, store the almonds in an airtight container for a crunchy, low-sugar treat.

Banana Oat Cookies:

Ingredients:

- 2 ripe bananas, mashed
- 1 1/2 cups rolled oats
- 1/4 cup chopped nuts (e.g., walnuts or almonds)
- 1/4 cup dark chocolate chips (optional)
- 1/2 teaspoon vanilla extract
- 1/2 teaspoon cinnamon

Instructions:

- Preheat your oven to 350°F (175°C).
- In a bowl, combine the mashed bananas, oats, nuts, dark chocolate chips (if using), vanilla extract, and cinnamon.
- Drop spoonfuls of the mixture onto a baking sheet lined with parchment paper.
- Bake for 15-20 minutes or until the cookies are golden brown.
- Allow them to cool before enjoying these naturally sweetened cookies.

Yogurt parfaits:

Ingredients:

- 1 cup of plain Greek yoghurt or your favourite yoghurt (for added probiotics, choose a yoghurt with live active cultures)
- 1/2 cup of granola (you can use store-bought or homemade granola)
- 1 cup of mixed berries (strawberries, blueberries, raspberries, or any fruit you prefer)
- 1-2 tablespoons of honey or maple syrup (optional, for sweetness)
- 1/4 cup of chopped nuts (e.g., almonds, walnuts, or pecans) for added crunch (optional)

Instructions:

1. Start by choosing a glass or a bowl for your parfait. Parfaits are often served in clear glasses to showcase their beautiful layers.
2. Begin with a layer of yoghurt at the bottom of your glass. You can sweeten the yoghurt with honey or maple syrup if desired.
3. Add a layer of granola on top of the yoghurt. The granola adds a delightful crunch and texture to the parfait.
4. Add a layer of mixed berries or the fruit of your choice on top of the granola. You can use fresh or frozen berries, but fresh berries are usually preferred for their texture and flavour.

5. If you'd like to add some nuts for extra crunch and a touch of healthy fats, sprinkle a layer of chopped nuts on top of the berries.

6. Repeat these layers until you reach the top of the glass or achieve the desired amount. Typically, a yoghurt parfait has 2-3 layers of yoghurt, granola, and fruit.

7. Finish with a drizzle of honey or maple syrup for extra sweetness if needed.

8. Optionally, garnish the top with a few whole berries or a mint leaf for presentation.

9. Serve your yoghurt parfait immediately or cover and refrigerate for a quick and convenient snack or breakfast option.

Variations:

- You can customize your yoghurt parfait by using different types of yoghurt (e.g., vanilla, coconut, or almond yoghurt) and fruits (e.g., mango, banana, or kiwi).

- Experiment with various granola flavours, such as cinnamon, almond, or chocolate chip.

- For a touch of indulgence, you can add a layer of chocolate chips, peanut butter, or Nutella.

- Consider adding chia seeds or flax seeds for extra fibre and omega-3 fatty acids.

Chapter 7: Beverages

Herbal teas and infusions:

Herbal Teas:

- Herbal teas are typically made from leaves, flowers, stems, or other plant parts that are steeped in hot water. They are often used for their pleasant taste and potential health benefits.

Recipe: Chamomile Tea

Ingredients:

- 1-2 teaspoons of dried chamomile flowers
- 8 oz (1 cup) of boiling water

Instructions:

1. Place the dried chamomile flowers in a tea infuser or a teapot.
2. Pour the boiling water over the chamomile.
3. Let it steep for 5-7 minutes.
4. Remove the infuser or strain the tea and enjoy.

Herbal Infusions:

- Herbal infusions are made by steeping larger amounts of plant material (usually leaves, flowers, or herbs) in hot water over an extended period, often several hours. This method extracts more flavour and nutrients.

Recipe: Mint Infusion

Ingredients:

- A handful of fresh mint leaves or 2-3 tablespoons of dried mint
- 8 oz (1 cup) of boiling water

Instructions:

1. Place the mint leaves in a teapot or a heatproof container.
2. Pour the boiling water over the mint.
3. Cover and let it steep for at least 15-20 minutes or longer for a stronger infusion.
4. Strain and serve.

Other Herbal Tea and Infusion Ideas:

Lavender Tea (Herbal Tea):

Ingredients:

- 1-2 teaspoons of dried lavender buds, 8 oz of boiling water.

Instructions:

- Steep lavender buds in boiling water for 5-7 minutes, strain, and enjoy the aromatic flavour.

Ginger and Lemon Infusion (Herbal Infusion):

Ingredients:

- Sliced fresh ginger, lemon slices, and 8 oz of boiling water.

Instructions:

- Combine ginger and lemon in a heatproof container, pour boiling water over them, steep for at least 20 minutes, strain, and sip this warming infusion.

Hibiscus Iced Tea (Herbal Tea):

Ingredients:

- Hibiscus petals, 8 oz of boiling water, sweetener (optional), ice cubes.

Instructions:

- Steep hibiscus petals in boiling water for 5-7 minutes, sweeten to taste (if desired) and chill with ice for a refreshing iced tea.

Nettle Infusion (Herbal Infusion):

Ingredients:

- Dried nettle leaves, 8 oz of boiling water.

Instructions:

- Steep dried nettle leaves in boiling water for several hours or even overnight for a nutrient-rich infusion.

Detox water recipes:

Lemon and Mint Detox Water:

Ingredients:

- 1 lemon, thinly sliced
- 10-12 fresh mint leaves
- 1.5 litres of water

Instructions:

1. In a large pitcher, add the lemon slices and mint leaves.
2. Fill the pitcher with water.
3. Refrigerate for a few hours to allow the flavours to infuse.
4. Serve chilled

Benefits: Lemon adds a burst of citrus flavour and provides vitamin C, while mint offers a refreshing taste. This combination is believed to aid digestion and boost metabolism.

Cucumber and Ginger Detox Water:

Ingredients:

- 1 cucumber, thinly sliced
- 1-inch piece of ginger, thinly sliced
- 1.5 litres of water

Instructions:

1. Place the cucumber slices and ginger in a pitcher.
2. Add water to the pitcher.
3. Let it chill in the fridge for a few hours before serving.

Benefits: Cucumber is hydrating and may reduce water retention, while ginger can help with digestion and add a spicy kick to the water.

Berry Blast Detox Water:

Ingredients:

- 1 cup of mixed berries (strawberries, blueberries, raspberries)
- 1.5 litres of water

Instructions:

1. Wash and rinse the berries.
2. Add the berries to a pitcher.
3. Pour water into the pitcher.
4. Let it sit in the refrigerator for a few hours to infuse the flavours.

Benefits: Berries are rich in antioxidants and can provide a burst of natural sweetness and colour to your water. They are believed to help detoxify the body and improve skin health.

Citrus and Cilantro Detox Water:

Ingredients:

- 2 oranges, thinly sliced
- 1 lime, thinly sliced
- A small handful of fresh cilantro
- 1.5 litres of water

Instructions:

1. Add the citrus slices and cilantro to a pitcher.
2. Fill the pitcher with water.
3. Allow it to infuse in the refrigerator before serving.

Benefits: Citrus fruits are a great source of vitamin C and add a zesty flavour. Cilantro provides a unique herbal twist to the water and is thought to help eliminate heavy metals from the body.

Smoothie ideas for cleansing:

1. Green Detox Smoothie:

- 1 cup of kale or spinach
- 1/2 cucumber
- 1/2 green apple
- 1/2 lemon, juiced
- 1-inch piece of ginger
- 1 cup of coconut water
- Ice cubes (optional)
- Blend all the ingredients until smooth.

2. Berry Antioxidant Smoothie:

- 1 cup of mixed berries (blueberries, strawberries, raspberries)
- 1/2 cup of spinach
- 1 tablespoon of chia seeds
- 1/2 cup of unsweetened almond milk
- 1 teaspoon of honey (optional)
- Ice cubes (optional)
- Blend all the ingredients until smooth.

3. Tropical Cleanse Smoothie:

- 1/2 cup of pineapple chunks
- 1/2 cup of mango chunks
- 1/2 banana
- 1 cup of coconut water
- 1 tablespoon of fresh lime juice
- 1 tablespoon of shredded coconut
- Ice cubes (optional)
- Blend all the ingredients until smooth.

4. Detoxifying Beet Smoothie:

- 1 small cooked beet, peeled and cubed
- 1/2 cup of frozen berries (e.g., raspberries, blueberries)
- 1/2 cup of spinach
- 1 tablespoon of flaxseed
- 1 cup of unsweetened almond milk
- Ice cubes (optional)
- Blend all the ingredients until smooth.

5. Cilantro and Cucumber Cleansing Smoothie:

- 1/2 cucumber
- 1/2 cup of fresh cilantro
- 1/2 lemon, juiced
- 1/2 lime, juiced
- 1 cup of coconut water
- 1 teaspoon of spirulina (optional)
- Ice cubes (optional)
- Blend all the ingredients until smooth.

Chapter 8: Meal Planning and Tips

How to plan lymphatic diet meals:

Meal planning for a lymphatic diet is selecting foods and substances that promote lymphatic system health and function. The lymphatic system is essential for the body's immune system and fluid homeostasis. Here's how to meal plan for a lymphatic diet:

1. **Consult with a Healthcare expert**: Before beginning any diet, consult with a healthcare expert, such as a qualified dietitian or nutritionist, to determine that the lymphatic diet is appropriate for your specific requirements and health objectives.

2. **Understand Lymphatic Diet concepts**: Become acquainted with the lymphatic diet concepts. This usually entails eating foods that are low in salt, high in antioxidants, anti-inflammatory, and beneficial to lymphatic drainage. Fruits, vegetables, lean meats, and whole grains are examples of these foods.

3. **Create a Balanced Plate:** Plan meals that incorporate a range of dietary categories. Aim for a platter that includes:

   - **Vegetables and fruits:** Make fruits and vegetables the foundation of your meals. They include a lot of antioxidants, vitamins, and minerals that help the lymphatic system. Colourful, leafy greens and cruciferous foods such as broccoli and cabbage should be prioritized.

- **Lean Proteins:** Include skinless poultry, fish, beans, and tofu as lean protein sources. Protein aids in the healing and maintenance of lymphatic tissues.

- **Whole Grains:** Choose whole grains such as quinoa, brown rice, and whole wheat bread for long-lasting energy and fibre.

- **Healthy Fats:** Include sources of healthy fats such as avocados, almonds, and olive oil in your diet. These fats promote general health and have the potential to decrease inflammation.

4. **Keep an eye on your sodium intake:** Sodium can lead to fluid retention, putting additional strain on the lymphatic system. Avoid highly processed meals, canned soups, and excessive salt use in cooking to reduce your sodium consumption.

5. **Stay Hydrated:** The lymphatic system requires enough water. To aid lymphatic drainage, drink lots of water throughout the day.

6. **Meal Control:** To avoid overeating, pay attention to meal proportions. Eating in moderation aids in weight maintenance and decreases the load on the lymphatic system.

7. **Include Healthy Snacks Between Meals**: Include healthy snacks between meals to maintain consistent energy levels and avoid overeating during main meals. Snacks can include fruits, veggies, nuts, and yoghurt.

8. **Include Lymphatic-Boosting Foods**: Include foods known to improve lymphatic health, such as ginger, garlic, turmeric, and antioxidant-rich foods like berries.

9. **Meal Preparation**: Consider meal preparation to have nutritional, lymphatic-friendly alternatives on hand. To save time, make salads, soups, and other items ahead of time.

10. **Monitor Your Progress**: Keep a food journal to chart your meals, and how your body reacts, and make changes as required.

11. **Consider Food Allergies and Sensitivities:** When preparing your meals, consider any food allergies or sensitivities you may have and find acceptable substitutions.

12. **Consult a Dietitian**: If you have special dietary limitations or health concerns, a trained dietitian may offer you individualized advice and meal planning that is suited to your unique requirements.

Grocery shopping for the diet:

Grocery shopping for the lymphatic diet involves selecting foods and ingredients that are supportive of a healthy lymphatic system.

1. **Fresh Fruits and Vegetables**: Focus on a variety of colourful fruits and vegetables. These are rich in vitamins, minerals, and antioxidants, which can help reduce inflammation and support lymphatic health. Look for options like berries, leafy greens, citrus fruits, and cruciferous vegetables.

2. **Lean Proteins**: Choose lean protein sources like skinless poultry, fish, lean cuts of beef or pork, and plant-based protein options such as tofu and legumes. Avoid processed meats, which tend to be high in sodium.

3. **Whole Grains**: Opt for whole grains like brown rice, quinoa, whole wheat pasta, and whole-grain bread. These provide complex carbohydrates, fibre, and nutrients.

4. **Low-Sodium Options**: Check food labels for sodium content and choose low-sodium or no-salt-added versions of canned goods like beans, tomatoes, and soups. Reducing sodium intake is important for a healthy lymphatic system.

5. **Healthy Fats**: Include sources of healthy fats, such as avocados, nuts, seeds, and olive oil. These fats can have anti-inflammatory properties.

6. **Dairy and Dairy Alternatives**: If you consume dairy, consider low-fat or fat-free options. For those following a

dairy-free diet, choose plant-based milk alternatives like almond, soy, or coconut milk.

7. **Herbs and Spices**: Stock up on herbs and spices like turmeric, ginger, garlic, and cinnamon. These can add flavour to your dishes and have anti-inflammatory properties.

8. **Nuts and Seeds**: Purchase a variety of nuts and seeds, such as almonds, walnuts, flaxseeds, and chia seeds. They can be used in salads, smoothies, and snacks.

9. **Low-Sugar and Natural Sweeteners**: When purchasing sweeteners, opt for natural options like honey, maple syrup, or stevia, and limit refined sugars.

10. **Beverages**: Focus on hydrating with water, herbal teas, and freshly squeezed juices. Minimize or avoid sugary and caffeinated beverages.

11. **Processed Foods and Snacks**: Minimize the purchase of processed foods, which are often high in sodium, sugar, and unhealthy fats. Instead, prepare homemade snacks with fresh ingredients.

12. **Allergen-Free Options**: If you have allergies or dietary restrictions, choose suitable alternatives. For example, if you're gluten-intolerant, look for gluten-free products.

13. **Organic and Non-GMO Options**: If possible and within your budget, consider selecting organic and non-genetically modified (non-GMO) products for a cleaner, chemical-free diet.

14. **Meal Planning**: Before you go shopping, plan your meals and create a list. This can help you avoid impulsive

purchases and stick to the foods that align with the lymphatic diet.

Tips for staying on track:

Staying on track with any diet plan, even the lymphatic diet, may be difficult. Here are some pointers to help you stick to your lymphatic diet:

1. **Meal Preparation**: Plan your meals and snacks ahead of time. This can help you ensure that you have the correct components on hand while also reducing the temptation to eat unhealthy foods.
2. **Keep Healthy Snacks on Hand:** Keep lymphatic-friendly foods and products in your pantry and refrigerator. When you're hungry in between meals, you'll have healthier alternatives at your disposal.
3. **Portion Control:** Be mindful of portion sizes. Excessive consumption of even nutritious meals might result in weight gain. If required, use measuring cups or a food scale.
4. Eating thoughtfully entails savouring each mouthful, eating carefully, and paying attention to your body's hunger and fullness signs. This might assist you in avoiding overeating.

5. **Stay Hydrated:** A healthy lymphatic system requires enough water. Stay hydrated throughout the day. To add variation, use lymphatic-friendly herbal teas or infused water.

6. **Variety is Important**: The lymphatic diet promotes a wide range of nutrient-dense foods. To make your meals interesting, try diverse fruits and vegetables, lean meats, and nutritious grains.

7. **Examine the Labels:** Keep an eye out for the components in packaged goods. Look for hidden sugars, excessive salt, and additives that may contradict the principles of the lymphatic diet.

8. **Reduce Your Consumption of Processed Foods:** Processed foods are generally heavy in salt, sugar, and harmful fats. Reduce your intake of processed and packaged foods.

9. **Include Exercise:** Physical exercise is beneficial to general health and can help the lymphatic system operate. Aim for frequent, enjoyable activities, such as walking, swimming, or yoga.

10. **Track Your Progress**: Maintain a food journal or use a diet monitoring app to record your meals and measure your progress. This might assist you in identifying areas for improvement.

11. **Seek Help:** Look for a support system, whether it's a buddy or an online group, where you can share your experiences, ask questions, and obtain inspiration.

12. **Treat Yourself:** It's fine to indulge in your favourite delicacies once in a while, as long as it doesn't become a habit. Moderation is essential.

13. **Consult an expert:** If you have special health problems or dietary requirements, consider speaking with a healthcare expert or certified dietitian who can give tailored advice.

Chapter 9: Conclusion

Accept Health and Feed Your Lymphatic System

As we near the end of the *"Lymphatic Diet Cookbook,"* I want to send you a message of hope, encouragement, and empowerment. Living with lymphatic problems might be difficult, but it does not have to define your life. You've gone on a journey of healing, sustenance, and self-discovery through the pages of this book.

We've looked at the fundamental relationship between what we eat and the health of our lymphatic system. You've heard about the tremendous benefits of nutrition, antioxidants, and water for lymphatic health. You've uncovered delectable recipes and meal ideas that will aid you on your wellness journey. However, the voyage does not finish here; rather, it is just beginning.

As a lymphatic patient, you have demonstrated amazing perseverance, courage, and tenacity. It's not always easy, but your dedication to your health is admirable. Remember that this cookbook is more than just a collection of recipes; it's a toolkit full of the resources you'll need to take charge of your health.

I urge you to embrace the joy of cooking and the beauty of nourishing your body when you close this book and enter your kitchen. Every meal you make from these pages is an act of self-love, a step toward greater health, and a commitment to yourself that you deserve to live the greatest life possible.

There will be difficulties, disappointments, and days when you feel defeated. But keep in mind that you are not alone. There is a whole community of people that understand your situation. Lean on them for encouragement, support, and inspiration. Share your experiences, successes, and even your vulnerable times. We can build a network of strength and knowledge that will empower every one of us.

The *"Lymphatic Diet Cookbook"* is your loyal friend, but keep in mind that it is only as excellent as the love and attention you put into it. Be kind to yourself, adjust recipes to your preferences and dietary constraints, and enjoy each meal as a gift to your body.

Your lymphatic system, like yours, deserves the finest. Allow this book to be your guide to restored health and vigour. Your path is distinct, and your tale is still being written. Accept it with all of your drive and elegance.

May each meal you create from this cookbook serve as a reminder of your great power. Your lymphatic system is on a rehabilitation and restoration trip, and you are its devoted guide.

Appreciate health, nourish your lymphatic system, and, most importantly, appreciate life's amazing adventure.

With love and optimism,

Vakarė Rimkutė